30 ORAL HYGIENE TIPS

Best Oral Hygiene Routines

By

Casey Armstrong

TABLE OF CONTENTS

Introduction

A healthy smile is not only aesthetically pleasing but it plays an essential role in preserving our overall wellbeing.

Healthy teeth and gums are built on a foundation of good oral hygiene, which also helps to prevent other dental problems including cavities, gum disease, and bad breath.

In this book, we will explore the greatest oral hygiene tips and important oral hygiene routines to help you maintain excellent dental health.

Understanding Oral Hygiene

The term "oral hygiene" refers to the customs and routines people follow to keep their mouths, teeth, and gums healthy.

Getting rid of plaque, bacteria, and food particles entails routine brushing, flossing, tongue cleansing, and other preventive treatments.

You can avoid dental issues, enhance your oral health, and promote a confident smile by maintaining appropriate oral hygiene.

The Importance of Oral Hygiene

For several reasons, maintaining proper dental hygiene is essential.

It helps in preventing tooth decay, which happens when oral bacteria produce acids that destroy the enamel on the teeth. Plaque, a sticky film of germs that builds up on teeth and promotes deterioration, is removed by regular brushing and flossing.

Gum disease is prevented by good dental hygiene. Periodontitis, a serious form of gum disease, can develop because of plaque and tartar accumulation along the gum line.

Bad breath caused by gaseous byproducts of the mouth bacteria is eliminated by practicing good dental hygiene.

Keeping up with good oral hygiene encourages general wellness. Numerous studies have discovered connections between poor dental health and several systemic diseases, including heart disease, respiratory infections, and unfavorable pregnancy outcomes. You can lower your risk of developing these issues by maintaining good dental health.

The following are oral hygiene tips that can help you achieve your desired result.

Tip 1: Brush Your Teeth At Least Twice a Day

It's crucial to brush your teeth at least twice a day to maintain proper oral hygiene and general health. Here are some justifications for why it matters:

Plaque removal:

Plaque, a sticky film of germs that accumulates on your teeth, is removed by brushing. If plaque is not effectively eliminated, it can cause gum disease, cavities, and tooth decay.

Food particle removal:

Regular tooth brushing helps to get rid of food particles that might lead to the production of acids. These substances can lead to enamel degradation and cause tooth decay.

Gum disease prevention:

Proper brushing can aid in the prevention of gum disorders including gingivitis and periodontitis. Plaque accumulation is what causes gum disease, which can result in bleeding and inflamed gums, foul breath, and tooth loss.

Fresh breath:

Brushing your teeth can help remove bacteria that cause bad breath in your mouth, giving you a more confident smile and fresher breath.

Preventing stains:

Brushing your teeth on a regular basis will help eliminate surface stains brought on by specific foods, beverages, and habits like smoking, keeping your smile bright.

Tip 2: Clean Your Tongue

To gently clean and eliminate bacteria from your tongue, use a tongue scraper or your toothbrush. A crucial component of maintaining proper dental hygiene is cleaning the tongue. Why it is crucial is as follows:

Removal of bacteria:

Food particles, dead cells, and bacteria all thrive on the surface of the tongue. By removing these collected bacteria, tongue cleaning helps to stop their growth and lowers the chance of developing foul breath (halitosis).

Prevention of oral diseases:

Tooth decay, gum disease, and oral infections can all be caused by bacteria on the tongue. You may lessen the number of bacteria in your mouth and minimize your risk of developing these diseases by frequently washing your tongue.

Fresher breath:

Removing the bacteria that cause foul breath by cleaning the tongue can assist. The back of the tongue, where bacteria can hide, is frequently the source of bad breath. Breath freshness can be considerably increased by routine tongue cleaning.

Improved appearance:

A clean tongue helps the mouth look cleaner. The appearance of your smile may be badly impacted by a coated or stained tongue. You can improve the overall appearance of your oral cavity by cleansing the tongue.

Tip 3: Floss Daily

Use dental floss or interdental brushes to remove plaque from between your teeth by flossing every day.

Daily flossing is essential for maintaining good dental hygiene. Several factors support the significance of flossing:

Removes plaque and debris:

Flossing reaches the areas between your teeth and along the gum line that a toothbrush cannot, removing plaque and other dirt there. Plaque, germs, and food particles that can assemble in these locations are removed with its assistance.

Prevents gum disease:

Gum disease can be avoided by avoiding plaque development, which can irritate and inflame the gums. By removing plaque from the gum line, flossing lowers the chance of developing periodontitis and gingivitis.

Reduces bad breath:

Food fragments stuck between teeth might exacerbate bad breath. By removing these impurities, flossing aids in breath freshening.

Improves total dental hygiene:

By completely cleaning surfaces that a toothbrush can't reach, flossing supports brushing. Your dental hygiene routine is complete, and total cleanliness is ensured.

Prevents tartar buildup:

Plaque can get hard and create tartar (calculus) on your teeth if it is not cleared away. Brushing and flossing alone are insufficient to eradicate tartar; professional dental cleaning is necessary. Regular flossing reduces the development of tartar.

Keep in mind that flossing correctly is crucial. Brush the spaces in between each tooth with an interdental brush or a piece of dental floss while gliding it softly up and down the sides.

Avoid snapping the floss against the gums to prevent harm. Alternatives like floss picks or water flossers may be helpful if you have trouble using regular floss.

To get the benefits and keep a healthy smile, make flossing a daily routine.

Tip 4: Use Mouthwash

Use mouthwash to get rid of bacteria and freshen your breath. Rinse your mouth out with an antibacterial mouthwash.

Including mouthwash in your oral care routine has many advantages. Here's why it's crucial:

Freshens breath:

By eradicating bacteria and neutralizing odor-producing substances in the mouth, mouthwash helps fight bad breath. It gives your breath a quick, fleeting boost in freshness.

Eliminates bacteria:

Mouthwash has antimicrobial components that can kill bacteria and lessen the number of bacteria in your mouth. By doing this, infections, gum disease, and tooth decay can all be avoided.

Reaches hard-to-brush areas:

Mouthwash can get to areas of the mouth that are challenging to reach with a toothbrush or floss. It can clean better since it may get in between teeth, along the gum line, and in other nooks and crannies.

Enhances plaque removal:

Mouthwash can improve plaque removal when used in conjunction with brushing and flossing. Overall oral hygiene can be improved by allowing it to loosen and remove plaque and any residual food particles.

Soothes oral tissues:

Oral tissues can be soothed and relieved by some of the substances included in mouthwashes. If you have minor mouth irritations, ulcers, or gum inflammation, this may be helpful.

Aids remineralization:

Remineralization is aided by fluoride, which is found in several types of mouthwash and helps to strengthen tooth enamel. This can offer defense against tooth decay and degradation of the enamel.

Promotes gum health:

Gum health is promoted using mouthwashes with antibacterial qualities, which can help lessen the bacterial load along the gumline, preventing gum disease, and enhancing gum health.

Provides an additional layer of protection:

Mouthwash can add another layer of defense against problems with oral health. By giving your oral hygiene efforts an extra boost, it enhances the benefits of brushing and flossing.

While mouthwash has some advantages, it shouldn't replace brushing and flossing.

Incorporate mouthwash into your regular oral care routine after consulting with your dentist to find the best option for your unique oral health requirements.

Tip 5: Replace Your Toothbrush Regularly

Every three to four months, or sooner if the bristles start to fray, you should replace your toothbrush or toothbrush head.

It's crucial to replace your toothbrush on a regular basis to maintain good oral hygiene. Here's why it's crucial:

Optimal bristle condition:

Over time, your toothbrush's bristles may fray, wear out, or become splayed. The toothbrush, therefore, loses some of its ability to effectively remove plaque and other particles from your teeth and gums. By replacing your toothbrush on a regular basis, you can make sure the bristles are in great shape for effective cleaning.

Bacterial buildup prevention:

Fungi, bacteria, and other microbes can live in toothbrushes. When you use an old toothbrush, these microorganisms can build up and multiply on the bristles, raising the possibility that you'll reinfect your mouth with dangerous bacteria. By switching out your toothbrush, you lower the likelihood of bacterial buildup and the danger of dental illnesses.

Gentle on gums:

Over time, wear and tear can cause toothbrush bristles to stiffen and become abrasive. Using a rough-bristled, old toothbrush can irritate your gums, causing swelling, irritation, and even gum recession. By regularly replacing your toothbrush, you can be sure that it has gentle, soft bristles that are good for your gums.

Preventing cross-contamination:

It's crucial to change your toothbrush after being sick or having a mouth infection. This aids in limiting the spread of any viruses or bacteria that could still be on the bristles.

It is advised to replace your toothbrush or toothbrush head every three to four months, or sooner if the bristles seem worn or splayed. Additionally, pay attention to any replacement-interval recommendations made by your dentist or the toothbrush manufacturer.

You can maintain the effectiveness of your oral hygiene practice and encourage the best oral health by routinely replacing your toothbrush.

Tip 6: Choose the Right Toothbrush

To gently reach every part of your mouth, choose a toothbrush with a tiny head and soft bristles.

A suitable toothbrush must be used to maintain good oral hygiene. Here are a few factors that make choosing the right toothbrush crucial:

Effective plaque removal:

Your teeth and gums can be cleaned of plaque, bacteria, and food particles with the correct toothbrush. To avoid tooth decay, gum disease, and other oral health problems, proper plaque removal is crucial.

Gentle on gums:

A toothbrush with soft bristles is kind to your gums and lowers your risk of gum sensitivity, recession, and irritation. The delicate gum tissue might be harmed by hard bristles that are too abrasive.

Proper size and shape:

The toothbrush head should have the right size and shape to easily reach all areas of your mouth, even difficult-to-reach areas like the rear molars. To successfully clean, it should fit comfortably and move around with ease.

Comfortable grip:

An ergonomic toothbrush is simpler to hold and manage while brushing. For those who suffer from arthritis or other disorders that impair hand dexterity, this is especially crucial.

Compatibility with your oral health needs:

Your specific oral health requirements should be considered while picking up a toothbrush. For instance, a toothbrush made for sensitive oral care may be helpful if you have sensitive teeth or gums.

Quality and durability:

Investing in a high-quality toothbrush ensures durability and longevity. A toothbrush with quality construction will perform better and endure longer.

For personalized advice on choosing the best toothbrush for your unique oral health requirements, speak with your dentist.

Tip 7: Brush at a 45-Degree Angle

For efficient plaque removal, hold your toothbrush at a 45-degree angle to your gum line.

An essential tip for good oral hygiene is to brush your teeth at a 45-degree angle. Here's why it's crucial:

Optimal plaque removal:

Brushing at a 45-degree angle enables the toothbrush bristles to reach the point where your teeth and gums converge. Plaque is prone to accumulating here, at the gum line.

You can successfully remove plaque from this important area by angling the brush, which lowers the risk of tooth decay and gum disease.

Gum stimulation:

Brushing at a 45-degree angle aids in enhancing gum health by stimulating the gums and improving blood flow. As a result, there may be less chance of gum disease and healthier gum tissue.

Effective tooth cleaning:

The bristles can reach the crevices between your teeth, where food particles and plaque can build up, thanks to the angled approach. The interdental areas are cleaned more effectively when brushed at a 45-degree angle, improving overall oral hygiene.

Gentle on the gums:

By brushing at a 45-degree angle, you make sure the bristles make contact with the gums as well as the teeth. It aids in the uniform distribution of pressure, reducing the possibility of gum irritation or injury. For keeping healthy gums and minimizing gum recession, gentle brushing is essential.

Proper reach:

Reaching all surfaces of the teeth, especially the rear molars, is possible by angling the toothbrush. This guarantees that you fully clean every area, leaving no stains unattended.

Stain removal:

Brushing your teeth at a 45-degree angle can also help remove surface stains. The bristles can efficiently scrape away stains brought on by meals, drinks, or behaviors like smoking since they can get into crevices.

Comprehensive cleaning:

Cleaning the gum line and tooth surfaces thoroughly is made possible by brushing at a 45-degree angle. It guarantees that you take care of both areas at once, giving you full cleaning experience.

Tip 8: Use Gentle Pressure When Brushing

When brushing, apply light pressure. Brushing too hard can harm your gums and tooth enamel.

To maintain good oral health, brushing your teeth with a light touch is essential. Here's why it's crucial:

Protects tooth enamel:

Brushing too vigorously might cause your teeth' enamel, which serves as a protective covering, to erode. dental discomfort, a higher risk of dental decay, and aesthetic problems like discolouration can all result from enamel degradation. Your enamel's integrity is preserved by applying light pressure.

Prevents gum injury:

Strenuous brushing with too much pressure can damage your gums, causing sensitivity, inflammation, and even gum disease. Applying little pressure prevents these problems and maintains the health of your gums.

Reduces toothbrush abrasion:

Too much force paired with the toothbrush bristles can damage the tooth structure, causing abrasion. This can eventually result in wear on the tooth surfaces or notches along the gumline.

You may lessen the chance of toothbrush abrasion and prolong the life of your teeth by brushing softly.

Allows proper cleaning technique:

Proper brushing technique is made possible by employing light pressure, which enables you to concentrate on making little circular or back-and-forth motions when brushing. It guarantees safe and efficient cleaning of the gum line and all tooth surfaces.

Promotes mindful brushing:

Applying light pressure motivates you to focus on your brushing technique and be conscious of the amount of pressure you use. By brushing with awareness, you can ensure thorough cleansing and be alert to any changes in your dental health, such as sensitivity or gum problems.

Brushing your teeth requires motion and not force. Apply light pressure with a soft-bristled toothbrush and let the bristles do the work. Concentrate on applying small, gentle motions to all tooth surfaces, including the gum line.

Tip 9: Brush Your Gum Line

To remove plaque and avert gum disease, gently brush along your gumline.

It is crucial to brush your teeth all the way down to your gum line to maintain good oral health. Here's why it's crucial:

Prevents gum disease:

Gum disease can be avoided by brushing the gum line, which helps get rid of plaque and bacteria that collect there. If this plaque isn't removed, it can cause gingivitis, an inflammation of the gums, which can develop into periodontitis, a more serious form of gum disease. Gum health is promoted, and the risk of gum disease is decreased by cleaning the gum line often.

Controls plaque buildup:

Plaque, a sticky bacterial film that builds regularly on your teeth and gums, can be reduced. Plaque can build up along the gum line and solidify into tartar (calculus), which is difficult to remove with just brushing. Plaque is disrupted and removed by brushing along the gum line, reducing tartar formation, and preserving a healthy dental environment.

Prevents gum recession:

Gum recession, in which the gums peel away from the teeth and expose the dental roots, is caused by neglecting the gum line. Plaque and bacteria that might cause gum recession are removed by brushing the gum line, preventing gum recession, and maintaining healthy gums.

Reduces bad breath:

Bad breath can be caused by bacteria that are found in plaque along the gum line. Reduce the bacterial load and the possibility of developing enduring foul breath by thoroughly cleansing the gum line.

Stimulates gum tissue:

Gum tissue is stimulated by brushing the gum line, which also increases blood flow to the gums and improves their general health. The gum tissue is kept robust, resilient, and less prone to inflammation thanks to this stimulation.

Enhances oral hygiene effectiveness:

The effectiveness of oral hygiene is increased by cleaning the gum line in addition to brushing the tooth surfaces. You can assure thorough plaque removal and lower your risk of cavities, gum disease, and other oral health problems by taking care of both the gum line and tooth surfaces.

It's crucial to remember that gum line bleeding or sensitivity could be an indication of gum disease or other oral health issues. It is advised in these situations to seek advice from your dentist or dental hygienist for a full analysis and customized recommendations.

Tip 10. Brush In a Circular Motion

Use circular motions to clean all tooth surfaces thoroughly.

Brushing in a circular motion is important for maintaining good oral hygiene and promoting overall dental health. Here are several reasons why brushing in a circular motion is beneficial:

Efficient plaque removal:

Brushing in a circular motion helps to effectively remove plaque from the teeth and gums. Plaque is a sticky film of bacteria that forms on the teeth and can lead to tooth decay and gum disease. Circular motions allow the bristles of the toothbrush to reach all areas of the teeth, including the spaces between them and along the gumline, ensuring a thorough cleaning.

Gentle on gums:

Brushing in a circular motion helps to minimize the risk of damaging the gums. Gentle circular motions distribute the pressure evenly, reducing the chances of gum irritation or abrasion. This technique is especially important for individuals with sensitive gums or those prone to gum recession.

Enhanced gum stimulation:

Circular brushing motions provide gentle stimulation to the gums, which can help improve blood circulation and promote gum health. Proper stimulation of the gum tissue can contribute to firmer and healthier gums, reducing the risk of gum problems such as gingivitis.

Complete coverage:

By brushing in a circular motion, you can ensure comprehensive coverage of all tooth surfaces. The circular motion helps reach areas that are often missed, such as the back teeth and the inner surfaces of the front teeth. This technique assists in removing food particles, bacteria, and plaque from all tooth surfaces, preventing cavities, and maintaining a clean mouth.

Improved control and technique:

Brushing in a circular motion offers better control and precision during brushing. This technique allows you to focus on each tooth individually, ensuring thorough cleaning and minimizing the chances of missing any areas. By brushing in small circles, you can effectively remove debris and plaque while maintaining proper brushing technique.

Tip 11: Don't Neglect Your Molars

Do not disregard your teeth: Since your rear teeth are more likely to get cavities, brush them more thoroughly.

To maintain proper oral hygiene and general dental health, it is essential to brush the molars or rear teeth. Here are a few explanations for why it's crucial to brush your molars:

Plaque and food removal:

Molars are more prone to plaque buildup and food debris because of their rough chewing surface and deep grooves and pits. Plaque, bacteria, and food particles that may become lodged in these difficult-to-reach places can be eliminated with the help of brushing the molars. You can stop cavities and tooth decay from developing by thoroughly cleaning the molars.

Prevention of gum disease:

Gum illnesses like gingivitis and periodontitis can develop because of failure to brush your molars, so be sure to do so. The accumulation of plaque on the molars can aggravate the gums, resulting in swelling and gum disease. The proper brushing of the molars encourages healthy gums by removing plaque, which can cause gum problems.

Protection against bad breath:

Molars, particularly the wisdom teeth at the rear of the mouth, are easily able to gather bacteria and food particles. If not removed by routine brushing, this dirt and bacteria can lead to bad breath. You may preserve fresh breath and avoid the formation of odor-causing chemicals by brushing your teeth carefully.

Tip 12: Wait to Brush after Acidic Foods

If you consume acidic meals or beverages, wait 30 minutes before cleaning your teeth to prevent enamel degradation.

For the sake of your oral health, brushing your teeth after consuming acidic meals or drinks is crucial. Here's why it's crucial:

Effects of acid neutralization:

Acidic foods and drinks, like citrus fruits, soda, and dressings made with vinegar, can temporarily soften the enamel on your teeth. After eating acidic foods, brushing your teeth can help neutralize the acid and reduce any potential damage to your tooth enamel.

Prevents loss of enamel:

Acidic substances can erode the enamel, the protective layer that covers your teeth. After consuming acidic foods, brushing your teeth helps remove any leftovers and shortens the time the acid is in touch with your teeth. This reduces the chance of enamel erosion, which can cause cavities, tooth sensitivity, and other dental issues.

Food residues are eliminated:

Acidic foods can leave behind little food residues or particles on your tongue. After consuming acidic foods, brushing your teeth helps eliminate these particles, keeping them from remaining in your mouth and promoting the growth of bacteria or foul breath.

Maintains fresh breath:

Foods and drinks that are acidic often leave you with a sour or unpleasant aftertaste. After eating, brushing your teeth helps to remove any remaining flavors or aromas brought on by acidic foods.

But you should avoid brushing your teeth for at least 30 minutes after consuming acidic meals or drinks. Acidic chemicals momentarily erode the enamel and brushing right away can exacerbate the problem. Instead, use water to rinse your mouth to help neutralize any acids after consuming acidic meals or beverages. Before brushing, you should wait to let your saliva naturally remineralize and reharden your tooth enamel.

Tip 13: Limit Sugary and Acidic Foods

Reduce your intake of sugary and acidic foods: Sugary and acidic foods might cause tooth decay.

To maintain proper oral hygiene and general dental health, sugary meals should be limited. Here's why it's crucial:

Prevention of tooth decay:

Sugar is a primary fuel for harmful bacteria in your mouth. The bacteria in your mouth feed on the sugar when you eat meals high in sugar, and therefore, the bacteria produce acids.

Your tooth enamel may be attacked and weakened by these acids, which can result in cavities and tooth decay. By reducing sugary foods, you lower the amount of fuel that bacteria have access to, lowering your risk of tooth decay.

Protection against gum disease:

Too much sugar consumption can potentially be a factor in the development of gum disease. When bacteria eat sugar, the resulting acids can irritate and inflame the gums, causing gingivitis and perhaps worsening gum disease. Sugary foods should be limited to preserve healthier gums and lower the chance of developing gum issues.

Preservation of tooth enamel:

Sugar can contribute to the demineralization of tooth enamel, particularly if it is consumed often throughout the day. Your teeth' protective layer becomes more vulnerable to damage and decay as a result of demineralization. Sugar consumption can be decreased while still maintaining the integrity and strength of dental enamel.

Balanced pH level in the mouth:

Sugary foods can make your mouth more acidic, which encourages the growth of dangerous germs. Limiting sugary meals will help you keep your mouth's pH level regulated, which is necessary for a healthy oral environment and the avoidance of gum disease and tooth decay.

It's crucial to remember that it's better to eat sugary foods in moderation and as a meal rather than as a solitary snack. This lessens how frequently sugar is consumed and how long your teeth are exposed to the acids that bacteria make.

Tip 14: Drink Water after Meals

Following a meal, sip some water to help rinse your mouth and balance acid levels.

It's good for your dental hygiene to drink water after eating. Here's why it's crucial:

Flushes away food particles:

Drinking water after meals aids in flushing away food particles that could be lodged in your teeth or around the gum line. Water functions as a natural cleanser, aiding in the removal of dirt and lowering the accumulation of bacteria and plaque.

Promotes saliva production:

Water encourages the production of saliva, which is necessary for maintaining a healthy mouth environment. Saliva assists in removing microorganisms and food particles from the mouth, neutralizing acids, and remineralizing teeth. After meals, drinking water stimulates saliva production, which improves dental health.

Maintains hydration:

Maintaining proper hydration is crucial for dental health as well as general well-being. After meals, drinking water keeps your mouth hydrated and helps avoid a dry mouth. Bad breath, tooth decay, and other oral health problems can all be influenced by a dry mouth. Maintaining proper hydration improves salivary gland health and contributes to a moist mouth environment.

Reduces acidity:

Water helps to dilute and neutralize the acids that are already present in your mouth after eating or drinking acidic foods or beverages. Water helps counteract the effects of acidic chemicals, which can momentarily erode tooth enamel and make teeth more sensitive.

Freshens breath:

Water can enhance your breath by washing away bacteria and leftover food particles that may cause bad breath. It gives your mouth a brief feeling of cleanliness and refreshment.

Tip 15: Avoid Smoking and Tobacco Use

Avoid smoking and using tobacco products: These behaviors raise your risk of oral cancer, tooth stains, gum disease, and tooth decay.

To maintain good oral hygiene and overall dental health, tobacco use should be avoided. This is why:

Increased risk of gum disease:

Smoking tobacco significantly increases the risk of developing gum disease (periodontal disease). It lessens blood supply to the gums, weakens the immune system, and delays recovery. Smokers are more likely to have tooth loss, have more severe symptoms of gum disease, and develop the condition.

Tooth discoloration:

Smoking stains teeth and over time can result in serious discolouration. Tobacco products' nicotine and tar stick to tooth enamel, leaving ugly yellow or brown stains. These stains can be challenging to get rid of with regular brushing and may need to be professionally cleaned or whitened.

Bad breath:

Smoking tobacco is a primary cause of this condition. Strong scents from tobacco products' ingredients might persist in the mouth, throat, and lungs. Smoking also causes a decrease in salivation, which can make bad breath worse.

Delayed healing after dental procedures:

The body's ability to heal and recuperate from dental treatments, such as tooth extraction, gum surgery, or dental implants, is impaired by smoking. It prolongs recovery time, slows down the healing process, and raises the possibility of problems.

Risk of oral cancer:

Oral cancer is significantly associated with tobacco use. Smokers are far more likely to acquire mouth, lip, tongue, throat, and other oral tissue malignancies. Tobacco products include dangerous compounds that can alter DNA and promote the development of malignant cells.

Reduced sense of taste and smell:

Smoking can impair one's ability to taste and smell, which makes it harder to properly appreciate food and beverages. Tobacco products contain compounds that can dull taste receptors and interfere with olfactory perception, making it difficult to recognize flavors and odors.

Increased plaque and tartar buildup:

Smoking encourages plaque buildup on teeth, which can result in the development of tartar (calculus). Plaque and tartar enable germs to flourish in an environment that raises the risk of gum disease, tooth decay, and other oral health issues.

Slower wound healing:

Smoking affects the delivery of oxygen and blood to tissues, particularly oral tissues. As a result, lesions like mouth sores, gum damage, or surgical incisions may take longer to heal.

The greatest course of action to safeguard your oral health and general well-being is to stop smoking. You can lower your risk of acquiring oral health issues and improve your oral hygiene by giving up smoking. For support and advice on how to successfully stop smoking, speak with your doctor or a smoking cessation professional.

Tip 16: Limit Your Alcohol Intake

Too much alcohol can cause dry mouth, foul breath, and a higher risk of oral cancer.

Alcohol use should be kept to a minimum to preserve dental health generally and proper oral hygiene. Here are a few explanations:

Dry mouth:

Alcohol is a diuretic, which means it increases urine production and can lead to dehydration. This causes dry mouth. Dry mouth, a condition where there is less saliva flow, can result from dehydration. Saliva is essential for maintaining good oral health because it washes away food residue, balances acidity, and inhibits bacterial growth. The likelihood of dental decay, gum disease, and foul breath are all increased by dry mouth.

Increased risk of oral cancer:

Oral cancer risk is increased by excessive alcohol use, which is a major risk factor. When paired with cigarette use, alcohol irritates oral tissues and dramatically raises the risk of oral cancer in the mouth, throat, and other parts of the oral cavity. Alcohol use should be kept to a minimum to lower the risk of mouth cancer.

Tooth erosion:

Many alcoholic beverages are acidic, which over time can destroy tooth enamel. Acidic beverages like wine, beer, and spirits erode the enamel's protective coating, leaving teeth more prone to damage and sensitivity. Alcohol use should be restricted both in terms of frequency and volume to reduce the risk of tooth erosion.

Staining and discoloration:

Alcoholic beverages can stain and discolor teeth, especially red wine and other dark alcoholic beverages like whiskey and coffee-based cocktails. Regular brushing can be difficult to eliminate these stains from the teeth, and professional dental cleaning or whitening procedures may be necessary.

Interference with wound healing:

Alcohol can impede the body's natural healing processes when it comes to wounds. Excessive alcohol use can impede your body's ability to heal after dental procedures like extractions, implants, or gum surgery and raise your risk of problems.

Increased risk of gum disease:

Alcohol can weaken the immune system and reduce the body's capacity to fight off diseases, including gum disease, which increases the chance of developing gum disease. The symptoms of gum disease, such as bleeding gums, gum recession, and tooth loss, can be brought on by excessive alcohol drinking.

It's crucial to remember that, if done safely and in moderation, moderate alcohol use may not significantly harm dental health. It is nevertheless advised to adopt appropriate oral hygiene practices and to be aware of any potential hazards.

Tip 17: Chew Sugar-Free Gum

Gum without sugar should be chewed after meals to increase salivation, which helps wash away food residue and neutralize acids.

Gum without sugar can be excellent for keeping your mouth healthy. Here's why it's crucial:

Stimulates saliva production:

Chewing sugar-free gum encourages saliva production. Saliva is produced in your mouth while you chew. Saliva aids in acid neutralization, the removal of food debris, and the remineralization of tooth enamel.

Increased saliva production encourages a healthy oral environment and can help fend off gum and tooth disease.

Cleanses the mouth:

Gum chewing helps to remove food particles and other debris from the teeth, gums, and other difficult-to-reach parts of the mouth. When you are unable to brush your teeth right away after a meal, this can be quite useful. After meals, chewing sugar-free gum for a short while can help remove leftover food and prevent plaque accumulation.

Neutralizes acids:

Acid neutralization: Xylitol, a component of sugar-free gum, can assist in neutralizing acids produced by oral bacteria. Chewing gum containing xylitol can help offset these effects and maintain a more balanced pH level in the mouth. Acidic environments contribute to tooth damage and erosion.

Reduces dry mouth symptoms:

Chewing gum increases saliva production, which is especially advantageous for people who suffer from xerostomia, or dry mouth. Bad breath, tooth decay, and other oral health problems can all be attributed to dry mouth. Sugar-free gum can temporarily relieve the symptoms of dry mouth by boosting salivation and moistening the oral tissues.

Freshens breath:

By disguising odors and lessening the effect of strongly scented foods or beverages, chewing sugar-free gum can help freshen your breath. It can contribute to a more pleasant oral environment and temporarily replace or supplement other breath-refreshing methods.

Tip 18: Stay Hydrated

Water is essential for maintaining saliva production and dental health throughout the day.

It's essential to stay hydrated to practice appropriate dental hygiene. Here's why it's crucial:

Production of saliva:

Proper hydration is necessary for the production of saliva, which is crucial for dental health. Saliva aids in lubricating the mouth, washing away food residue, and balancing bacterial acidity. Maintaining a healthy oral environment and avoiding problems like dry mouth, tooth decay, and gum disease require adequate saliva flow.

Prevention of dry mouth:

Xerostomia, a disease when the salivary glands do not generate enough saliva, can result from dehydration. A dry mouth can be uncomfortable, make it harder to speak and swallow, and raise your risk of developing oral health issues. Staying hydrated keeps the salivary glands functioning properly and helps avoid a dry mouth.

Oral tissue health:

Hydration is crucial for preserving the condition of oral tissues, such as the mucous membranes, tongue, and gums. These tissues acquire a suitable amount of oxygen and nutrients when they are well-hydrated, which improves their general health and lowers their vulnerability to infections and sores.

Acid neutralization:

Water consumption supports a healthy pH balance in the mouth, preventing the formation of an acidic environment that can erode tooth enamel and cause dental decay.

To prevent tooth decay, water can help dilute and neutralize acids created by bacteria and acidic foods and beverages.

Flushing away debris:

Drinking water throughout the day aids in rinsing away debris from the teeth and gums, including food particles, bacteria, and plaque. It functions as a natural cleaner, fostering good oral hygiene and lowering the likelihood of dental issues.

Freshens breath:

Avoiding dehydration can help you have better breath. Halitosis (bad breath) can be exacerbated by dry mouth, which can result from dehydration. You may lessen the symptoms of a dry mouth and retain fresher breath by keeping up a healthy water level.

Tip 19: Avoid Chewing on Ice, Hard Candies, or Objects

Avoid chewing on hard objects, ice, or candy because these behaviors might break or chip your teeth.

It's crucial to refrain from chewing on hard sweets, ice, or other objects to keep your mouth healthy. Here's why it's crucial:

Tooth damage:

Putting too much pressure on your teeth when you chew on ice, hard candies, or other things increases the chance of tooth injury. These behaviors may result in tooth fractures, chips, or cracks that may need dental work to fix. Damaged teeth are more prone to dental decay and other issues with oral health.

Enamel erosion:

Sugar is frequently used in the production of ice and hard candies, and prolonged contact with sugary things can cause enamel erosion. Sugar-feeding oral bacteria create acids, which over time may erode tooth enamel. The teeth become more prone to decay, sensitivity, and discolouration because of enamel erosion.

Chewing on hard items can cause jaw muscle strain, which can result in temporomandibular joint (TMJ) problems. Pain, discomfort, and trouble moving the jaw are all possible effects of TMJ issues. These problems can be avoided by avoiding practices that put an excessive amount of stress on the jaw.

Increased sensitivity of the teeth:

Chewing on hard things can wear away the enamel's protective coating, exposing the dentin beneath, which has sensitive nerve endings. As a result, eating or drinking things that are hot, cold, or sweet may cause pain or discomfort in the teeth.

Oral injuries:

The danger of mouth injuries increases while chewing on harsh things. Biting down firmly on ice or hard candies can result in tongue injuries, lacerations, wounds, or other soft tissue damage. These wounds may hurt and necessitate medical attention.

Dental work complications:

Chewing on hard items can harm fillings, crowns, or veneers that have been placed. These restorations may fracture or come loose when you bite down on ice or hard candies, necessitating extra dental work to fix or replace them.

Oral health complications:

Chewing on hard items can upset the normal balance of oral flora, which can lead to gum disease, foul breath, and mouth infections. Hard objects' jagged edges or uneven surfaces can harbor bacteria as well, making thorough tooth cleaning more difficult.

It is important to refrain from chewing on ice, hard candies, or other objects to safeguard your teeth and maintain proper dental hygiene. Choose healthy substitutes instead, such as sugar-free gum or mints, which can offer comparable mouth stimulation without the dangers of hard items. It is advised to seek professional assistance if you chew on non-food items frequently to address the root causes and choose healthier substitutes.

You can safeguard your teeth, keep up a healthy smile, and avoid needless dental issues by refraining from bad chewing habits.

Tip 20: Use Fluoride Toothpaste

Use fluoride toothpaste to help prevent cavities and improve tooth enamel.

It is essential to use fluoride toothpaste to maintain proper dental hygiene. Here's why it's crucial:

Strengthens tooth enamel:

Fluoride is a mineral that contributes to the strengthening of tooth enamel, the outer protective coating of the teeth. Remineralizing weak spots in the enamel strengthens them so they can withstand acid attacks from bacteria and carbohydrates. By adding additional protection to the teeth, regular use of fluoride toothpaste helps prevent tooth decay and cavities.

Prevents tooth decay:

Fluoride toothpaste has a great deal of success in preventing tooth decay. It aids in preventing the development of oral bacteria and lessens their capacity to create acids that can erode tooth enamel. You may dramatically lower your risk of getting cavities and keep your smile healthier by using fluoride toothpaste.

Remineralizes early-stage tooth decay:

Fluoride has the power to stop tooth decay in its tracks. Fluoride can help remineralize and strengthen the weakened portions of enamel that have started to demineralize, stopping the decay from spreading further. The early diagnosis and reversal of tooth decay can be helped by using fluoride toothpaste on a regular basis.

Protects against acid erosion:

Fluoride can assist in protecting teeth from acid erosion brought on by acidic foods, beverages, and oral environments. It fortifies the enamel, increasing its resistance to acid's erosive effects. By using fluoride toothpaste, you can reduce acid erosion and maintain the health of your teeth.

Suitable for all ages:

Fluoride toothpaste is appropriate for people of all ages, including adults and small children. Fluoride toothpaste is especially beneficial for children because their developing teeth are more susceptible to decay. To avoid consuming too much fluoride, it's crucial to use fluoride toothpaste that is appropriate for children's age.

You may strengthen your tooth enamel, avoid tooth decay, and have a healthy smile by integrating fluoride toothpaste into your daily oral care regimen.

Tip 21: Visit Your Dentist Regularly

For optimum oral health, schedule routine dental cleanings and exams every six months.

Regular dental visits are necessary to keep up good oral hygiene. Here's why it's crucial:

Professional dental cleaning:

When you visit the dentist regularly, dental professionals may thoroughly clean your teeth, removing plaque and tartar buildup that normal brushing and flossing cannot successfully eliminate. Professional cleanings aid in the prevention of tooth decay, gum disease, and other oral health issues.

Early dental problem detection:

Routine dental examinations allow for the early identification of dental concerns such as cavities, gum disease, oral infections, and oral cancer. Dentists are equipped with the knowledge and skills necessary to recognize and diagnose these problems when they are still relatively simple to resolve. Early treatment can stop dental issues from getting worse and spare you from needing future, more involved, and expensive procedures.

Oral cancer screening:

During routine dental visits, dentists check patients for mouth cancer. Early oral cancer detection considerably increases the likelihood of successful therapy. A quick identification of any worrisome lesions or anomalies in the oral tissues is made possible by routine dental checkups, enhancing the likelihood of an early diagnosis and favorable treatment results.

Personalized oral health advice:

Dental professionals offer insightful counsel and individualized suggestions for preserving excellent oral health. They may address your unique oral health issues, offer guidance on proper brushing and flossing techniques, suggest appropriate oral hygiene products, and give you suggestions on how to make your oral hygiene practice better. You can adequately take care of your teeth and gums at home with the help of this advice.

Preventive treatments:

During your routine checkups, the dentist might do preventive procedures. These may consist of fluoride treatments, dental sealants, and other preventive methods that help shield your teeth against decay, enamel erosion, and other dental problems. Children and those with an increased risk of dental issues may benefit most from these procedures.

Dental health monitoring:

Through routine checkups, your dentist can keep track of the condition of your teeth, gums, and oral tissues. They can keep tabs on any alterations or patterns and spot potential danger indicators or early indications of oral issues. Your dentist can offer the proper interventions and advice to maintain or improve your oral hygiene by keeping an eye on your dental health.

Evaluation of general health:

There is a strong relationship between oral and general health. Dentists can evaluate your general health during routine dental visits and look for any mouth symptoms of underlying illnesses or problems. Gum disease and other oral health disorders can exacerbate systemic health conditions like diabetes and cardiovascular disease. Dentists can improve your general health by addressing issues with your oral hygiene.

Regular checkups and cleanings at the dentist should be done every six months, on average. However, the frequency may change based on your dental health requirements and the advice of your dentist. Keep in mind that routine dental checkups support your daily oral hygiene routine and contribute to the long-term health of your teeth, gums, and entire oral cavity.

Regular dental appointments allow you to monitor your oral health, identify and address issues as they arise, get expert advice, and take advantage of a healthy, attractive smile.

Tip 22: Avoid Using Your Teeth as Tools

Don't use your teeth as a tool to open bottles or packages; doing so might cause chips or fractures.

It's crucial to refrain from using our teeth as implements to practice appropriate dental hygiene. This is why it is essential:

Prevents tooth damage:

Using our teeth as tools by biting or tearing things might seriously harm our teeth. The purpose of teeth is to chew food, not to rip open packages or shatter nuts. Too much force or using our teeth on objects that aren't food might chip or break teeth, which may necessitate costly dental work.

Reduces the risk of tooth sensitivity:

The enamel that covers our teeth protects the delicate inner layers from outside stimuli. But using our teeth as tools can erode the enamel and reveal the dentin below. Increased tooth sensitivity may result from this, making it painful or uncomfortable to consume hot, cold, or sweet foods and beverages.

Reduces the likelihood of developing jaw joint issues:

The temporomandibular joint (TMJ), which joins the jawbone to the skull, can experience excessive strain when teeth are used for purposes for which they were not designed. The TMJ can get stressed from repetitive or vigorous motions like opening bottle lids or shredding hard packaging, which can lead to jaw joint issues like pain, clicking, or difficulties moving the jaw.

Prevents oral infections:

Using our teeth as instruments increases the risk of oral infections by introducing foreign objects or substances into our mouths. Oral infections, gum disease, or even systemic illnesses can result from biting or tearing objects that may be filthy, polluted, or contaminated with germs. It is advisable to use the proper equipment and refrain from putting anything that could be hazardous in our mouths.

Preserves dental restorations:

Using your teeth as tools might harm or dislodge dental restorations like fillings, crowns, or veneers. Dental restorations are not intended to be used for purposes other than eating; they are only made to endure the forces of typical chewing and biting. The integrity and durability of your dental restorations are preserved when you refrain from using your teeth as instruments.

Promotes proper oral hygiene:

Using our teeth as implements can obstruct our oral hygiene routines. For instance, using our teeth to open bottles may result in wounds that make it difficult to effectively brush or floss. Additionally, improper tooth use increases the risk of gum disease and tooth decay by introducing bacteria or debris into the gum line. Maintaining good oral health requires practicing good oral hygiene and employing the right tools for non-oral duties.

It's critical to keep in mind how priceless and irreplaceable our teeth are. They are not intended to serve multiple purposes but rather for biting, chewing, and speaking. We may maintain the strength, functionality, and general health of our teeth by using the proper instruments for different tasks and avoiding the improper use of our teeth.

Tip 23: Rinse Your Toothbrush after Use

Your toothbrush should be properly rinsed after each use, and you should store it upright to let it air dry.

It's crucial to rinse our toothbrushes after each usage to maintain healthy oral hygiene. This is why it is essential:

Removes residual toothpaste and debris:

Rinsing our toothbrush after use helps to eliminate any leftover toothpaste, saliva, and food fragments that might have been left on the bristles.

This keeps bacteria from growing and guarantees that the toothbrush is clean and ready for use again.

Prevents bacterial development:

Moist conditions are favorable for bacterial growth, and a moist toothbrush can turn into a bacterial spawning ground. After each usage, we should thoroughly rinse our toothbrush to help eliminate moisture and reduce the formation of bacteria on the bristles.

Lowers the possibility of cross-contamination:

Rinsing our toothbrush reduces the likelihood of cross-contamination. Rinsing your toothbrush after use can help prevent the spread of germs, viruses, or other pathogens if several toothbrushes are kept together or near one another.

Maintains bristle effectiveness:

As toothpaste and other substances build up on the bristles, our teeth, and gums can become less effectively cleaned. To get the best brushing results, the toothbrush should be rinsed frequently to keep the bristles clean and free of buildup.

Prevents the growth of mold or mildew:

A toothbrush can promote the growth of mold or mildew if it is not thoroughly cleaned and allowed to dry. After usage, thoroughly rinsing the toothbrush and letting it air dry can help stop the growth of these undesirable germs.

Holding your toothbrush under running water for a brief period will guarantee that it has been well-rinsed. Shake off the excess water after rinsing, then store the toothbrush upright so that it may air dry in between uses. Brushes should not be covered or kept in closed containers as this can encourage bacterial growth.

You may maintain a clean and hygienic oral care regimen, ensuring the efficacy of your brushing efforts, and encouraging good oral health by implementing the practice of washing your toothbrush after each use.

Tip 24: Don't Share Toothbrushes

Avoid sharing toothbrushes: Doing so increases the risk of infection and the transmission of bacteria.

To maintain good oral hygiene, it's crucial to avoid sharing toothbrushes. This is why it is essential:

Bacterial transmission:

The sharing of toothbrushes can result in the spread of germs and other microbes between people. Sharing toothbrushes can bring alien bacteria into the mouth, raising the risk of infections, gum disease, and other oral health issues. Everyone has a different oral microbiome.

Viral and fungal infections:

Infections caused by viruses and fungi: Some viral and fungi infections are easily disseminated by saliva and oral contact. These diseases, such as oral thrush (Candida fungus), cold sores (herpes simplex virus), and other contagious oral illnesses, can spread more easily when toothbrushes are shared.

Bloodborne pathogens:

Sharing a toothbrush can put you at danger of spreading bloodborne pathogens if it has come into contact with blood, as is the case with bleeding gums or oral injuries. This is especially important when toothbrushes are shared among family members or when appropriate sterilization is not feasible.

Personal hygiene practices:

A single person should only use a toothbrush because it is a personal hygiene item. Sharing toothbrushes can damage oral hygiene regimens and impair personal hygiene behaviors. Sharing can undermine the customized aspect of oral hygiene because each person's toothbrush is designed to meet their unique needs for oral health.

Cross-contamination:

When toothbrushes are shared, oral bacteria, viruses, and other pathogens may spread. It is still possible to carry and spread dangerous bacteria that can affect oral health even if there are no outward symptoms of disease or infection. Cross-contamination is reduced to a minimum by not sharing toothbrushes.

Personal hygiene habits:

Maintaining good hygiene standards can be challenging when toothbrushes are shared. It may be difficult to remember which toothbrush belongs to whom, which could cause confusion and possible mix-ups. To guarantee good hygiene and avoid accidental sharing, each person needs their own toothbrush that is carefully labeled and preserved.

Long-term oral health:

Consistently practicing proper oral hygiene is crucial. You can remove plaque, avoid tooth decay and gum disease, and keep your mouth healthy by using your own toothbrush and practicing good oral hygiene. These efforts may be compromised if toothbrushes are shared, and oral health problems may result.

Use your own toothbrush and avoid sharing it with anybody else to maintain proper oral hygiene and reduce the risk of problems and infections. Each person needs their own toothbrush, which should be stored properly and updated on a regular basis. Encourage people to adopt the same hygiene practices and inform them of the dangers that could arise from sharing toothbrushes.

Tip 25: Limit Caffeine Consumption

Excessive caffeine intake can cause teeth grinding (bruxism) and stain your teeth.

Limiting caffeine consumption can be beneficial for maintaining good oral hygiene. Here's why it is important:

Staining of teeth:

Caffeinated beverages like coffee, tea, and certain sodas can cause staining of the teeth over time. The dark pigments in these drinks, such as tannins in tea and coffee, can adhere to the enamel, resulting in yellowing or discoloration of the teeth. Limiting caffeine consumption helps minimize the risk of dental staining and helps maintain a brighter smile.

Tooth enamel erosion:

Some caffeinated beverages, such as energy drinks and certain sodas, are highly acidic. Acidic drinks can gradually erode the protective enamel layer of the teeth, making them more susceptible to tooth decay and sensitivity. By reducing caffeine intake, you can minimize the exposure of your teeth to these acidic substances and help preserve the integrity of your tooth enamel.

Dry mouth:

Caffeine has diuretic properties, which means it can increase urine production and potentially lead to dehydration.

Dehydration can contribute to dry mouth, a condition characterized by reduced saliva production. Saliva plays a crucial role in oral health by neutralizing acids, washing away food particles, and helping to prevent tooth decay.

Limiting caffeine consumption helps maintain proper hydration and supports healthy saliva production, reducing the risk of dry mouth and its associated oral health issues.

Increased risk of bruxism:

Caffeine consumption has been linked to an increased risk of bruxism, which is the grinding or clenching of teeth, often during sleep. Bruxism can lead to tooth wear, jaw pain, headaches, and other dental problems. By limiting caffeine intake, especially in the evening, you can help reduce the likelihood of developing bruxism and minimize its impact on your oral health.

Better hydration choices:

Reducing caffeine consumption allows for greater consumption of water and other non-caffeinated, hydrating beverages. Water is essential for maintaining optimal oral health as it helps to rinse away food particles, stimulate saliva production, and maintain a moist environment in the mouth. Choosing hydrating alternatives to caffeinated beverages supports better overall oral hygiene.

Remember, moderation is key. If you choose to consume caffeinated beverages, consider drinking them through a straw to minimize contact with the teeth, rinse your mouth with water afterward, and maintain a consistent oral hygiene routine of brushing twice a day and flossing daily.

By limiting caffeine consumption, you can help protect your teeth from staining, preserve tooth enamel, maintain proper hydration and saliva production, reduce the risk of bruxism, and promote overall oral health.

Tip 26: Use a Straw for Sugary or Acidic Drinks

When consuming sugary or acidic beverages, use a straw to reduce direct contact between the liquid and your teeth.

For drinks that are sweet or acidic, using a straw can help you to maintain good dental hygiene. Here's why it's crucial:

Reduces direct contact:

Using a straw, especially one that is positioned in the back of your mouth, can reduce the amount of time that sugary or acidic beverages come into direct touch with your teeth. As a result, less dangerous substances—such as carbohydrates, acids, and pigments—that might cause tooth decay, enamel erosion, and staining are exposed to your tooth enamel.

Lowering the chance of dental decay:

Sugary drinks, such as soda, fruit juices, and energy drinks, can act as a feeding supply for oral bacteria. Byproducts from these bacteria include acids, which can attack tooth enamel and cause tooth decay. By avoiding direct contact between these beverages and your teeth by using a straw, you can help prevent tooth decay and maintain your oral health.

Protects tooth enamel:

Acidic beverages can damage your teeth's protective enamel layer, including citrus juices, sports drinks, and some sodas. As a result, the teeth may become weaker and more prone to sensitivity and cavities. By allowing the acidic beverage to avoid the surfaces of your teeth, using a straw helps to prevent enamel erosion and maintain the strength of your dental enamel.

Limits staining:

Over time, dark-colored drinks including coffee, tea, red wine, and some sodas can stain teeth. You can lessen the risk of staining and preserve a whiter smile by using a straw that is positioned toward the rear of your mouth to help prevent direct contact between these drinks and the front surfaces of your teeth.

Promotes better oral hygiene habits:

The use of a straw when drinking sweet or acidic beverages encourages better oral hygiene practices. When you drink through a straw, you might naturally be more likely to brush your teeth or rinse your mouth out with water afterward to lessen the harm that these beverages do to your teeth. This encourages preventative dental care and aids in maintaining better overall oral hygiene.

Always remember to select a straw that is suitable for the beverage you are drinking. Choose reusable or environmentally friendly ones, and take care to clean and maintain your straw properly to prevent bacterial growth.

When drinking sugary or acidic beverages, using a straw can help prevent tooth disease, erosion of the enamel, and discoloration. It encourages improved oral hygiene practices, supports overall oral health, and permits you to partake in your preferred beverages with a lower chance of tooth damage.

Tip 27: Avoid Excessive Teeth Whitening

Over-whitening your teeth might harm your tooth enamel and cause discomfort.

Maintaining good dental hygiene and protecting the health of your teeth requires avoiding over-bleaching. Here's why it's essential:

Tooth sensitivity:

Tooth sensitivity may be exacerbated by overly aggressive teeth-whitening procedures. Because of the temporary weakening of the enamel caused by the bleaching agents in whitening treatments, teeth may become more sensitive to hot, cold, and acidic foods and beverages. Longer or more frequent whitening sessions may make this sensitivity worse and hurt.

Gum irritation:

Overusing or applying tooth whitening treatments incorrectly might irritate the gums. When bleaching substances come into touch with delicate tissues, it can cause chemical burns, gum inflammation, and irritation. To reduce the danger of gum inflammation, it is crucial to adhere to the directions given by dental specialists or product manufacturers.

Enamel erosion:

Some tooth whitening solutions, particularly those that contain abrasives, may be responsible for this condition. Excessive or harsh bleaching can gradually remove the enamel's protective covering, leaving the teeth more susceptible to decay, sensitivity, and discolouration. It's crucial to follow the instructions on teeth-whitening products and seek the advice of a dentist for specific recommendations.

Uneven whitening:

Too much teeth whitening might produce blotchy or uneven whitening results. The teeth may overly whiten some places over time while leaving others unchanged. This may result in an unnatural appearance and the need for extra dental work to fix it.

Weakened tooth structure:

Too much usage of teeth-whitening products, particularly those with high bleaching chemical concentrations, might weaken the tooth structure. The teeth's general health and longevity may be compromised due to an increase in the possibility of fractures or other types of injury.

Before beginning any teeth-whitening treatment, it's crucial to speak with a dental practitioner. They may evaluate the state of your teeth, choose the best whitening methods for you, and offer advice on how frequently and how long the procedure should last. Under their supervision, expert dental cleanings and whitening procedures may assist guarantee outcomes that are both secure and efficient.

If you want a brighter smile, think about using natural treatments or less aggressive whitening products.

Always put your teeth's general health and integrity first.

Tip 28: Massage Your Gums

Gently massage your gums with your fingertips to increase blood flow and support gum health.

Gum massage is crucial to maintaining good dental hygiene. Here are some advantages:

Improved blood circulation:

Circulation is improved thanks to gum massage, which encourages blood flow to the gum tissues. The gums receive vital nutrients and oxygen from the improved circulation, which supports the gums' overall health and the healing process.

Strengthened gum tissues:

Regular gum massage might help to make the gum tissues stronger. It promotes the growth of a solid and hardy gum line, which can guard the teeth and stop gum recession.

Reduced inflammation:

Massaging the gums might aid in reducing edema and inflammation in the gum tissues. For people with gingivitis, an early stage of gum disease characterized by redness, soreness, and inflammation of the gums, it may be very helpful.

Improved gum health:

Massaging the gums can assist with clearing the gum line of bacteria and plaque. You can lessen your risk of developing gum disease and promote healthier gums by gently applying pressure to release any debris or germs that may be lodged along the gum border.

Improved oral hygiene:

Gum massage can enhance your daily oral hygiene regimen. You can do it gently and circularly with a clean finger or a toothbrush with soft bristles. By removing plaque and food particles, this movement increases the efficiency of brushing and flossing.

Reduced gum sensitivity:

Gum sensitivity can be lessened by gum massage. It may have a calming effect and desensitize the gum tissues, reducing their sensitivity to pain or discomfort.

Relaxation and stress relief:

Gum massage can be calming and relieving. Gum nerve endings are stimulated by massaging them, which helps people feel peaceful and at ease.

It's crucial to remember that a gentle, clean hand or a toothbrush with a soft bristle should be used when massaging the gums. A harsh method or excessive pressure should be avoided since these can irritate or harm the gums. It is advised to get advice from a dental expert for an assessment if you feel ongoing gum discomfort, bleeding, or any other unsettling signs.

Gum massage can benefit your oral health in many ways, including healthier gums, better blood flow, less inflammation, and better-looking teeth. It is an easy and helpful procedure that may be done on a regular basis to promote the health of your gums and teeth.

Tip 29: Consider Dental Sealants

Take dental sealants, which are thin coatings used to protect teeth on chewing surfaces against cavities in both children and adults.

For toddlers and teenagers in particular, dental sealants should be taken into consideration to preserve good oral health. Here's why they're advantageous:

Protection against cavities:

Dental sealants, which are thin, protective coatings placed on the chewing surfaces of the rear teeth (molars and premolars), provide protection against cavities. The deep grooves and crevices that food particles and germs can easily get stuck in and cause cavities are blocked off by them, acting as a barrier. Sealants give an extra layer of defense, lowering the chance of tooth decay.

Prevention of early tooth loss:

One of the main factors contributing to early tooth loss in children is tooth decay. Applying dental sealants considerably lowers the risk of acquiring cavities, preserving natural teeth, and avoiding early tooth loss.

Easy and painless application:

Dental sealants are placed easily and without any discomfort. After properly cleaning the teeth, the chewing surfaces are painted with a thin coat of dental sealant substance. After being subjected to a specific laser to harden it, the material forms a sturdy and protective barrier over the teeth.

Long-lasting protection:

Dental sealants offer ongoing protection against cavities for several years. The sealants will remain intact and functional with regular dental checkups. To ensure their durability, they can be fixed or applied again if necessary.

Cost-effective preventive measure:

Dental sealants are a preventive intervention that is both affordable and effective. The placement of sealants on the permanent molars and premolars can help avoid the need for future, more involved, and pricey dental procedures like fillings or crowns.

Improved oral hygiene outcomes:

Cleaning the teeth is made simpler by dental sealants. Brushing is more efficient in removing plaque and food particles from chewing surfaces because of the smooth surface that the sealants provide. This encourages improved dental care and lowers the chance of tooth decay.

Safe and non-invasive procedure:

The application of dental sealants is a safe and non-invasive procedure. Drilling or removing tooth structure is not necessary. Most people tolerate sealants well, and there are no substantial dangers or adverse effects associated with using them.

Suitable for all ages:

Although dental sealants are frequently applied to children and teenagers, adults who are more likely to get cavities may also benefit from them. Adults who have teeth with deep cracks or grooves can benefit from sealants to keep their teeth healthy and prevent decay.

It's crucial to remember that regular brushing, flossing, and dental exams go hand in hand with dental sealants. They add an additional layer of defense but do not take the place of proper oral hygiene habits.

To ascertain whether dental sealants are suitable for you or your child, speak with a dental expert. They can evaluate your dental health and suggest sealants as a part of a thorough preventive strategy for preserving excellent oral health.

Tip 30: Treat Dental Problems Promptly

Immediately seek dental care if you feel tooth pain, sensitivity, or any other oral health problems to avoid additional troubles.

For the sake of maintaining good oral health and avoiding further consequences, dental issues must be treated right away. Here's why it's crucial:

Pain and discomfort reduction:

Dental issues including tooth decay, gum disease, or infections can be quite painful and uncomfortable. By getting treatment right away, you can take care of the discomfort and stop it from getting worse, restoring your comfort, and enabling you to go about your everyday activities.

Preservation of natural teeth:

Prompt treatment might help you keep your natural teeth. Untreated dental problems might worsen and necessitate more involved procedures like extractions or root canals, tooth loss, or both. You maximize your chances of keeping your natural teeth and avoiding invasive operations by taking care of dental issues as soon as they arise.

Prevention of further complications:

Dental issues might result in more serious complications if not corrected. For instance, unattended tooth decay can develop into an infection that spreads to the jawbone, the surrounding tissues, or even other body parts. Prompt dental care can help stop the emergence of more sophisticated, perhaps dangerous problems.

Reduced treatment complexity and cost:

Early intervention frequently entails simpler and less expensive treatments. Early dental disorders that are identified and treated often call for less invasive procedures and have lower treatment costs. Delaying therapy could result in the condition getting worse and requiring more involved, time-consuming, and expensive operations.

Preserved oral function:

Dental issues might impair your capacity to chew and speak normally. If you receive prompt treatment, your oral function can be restored, allowing you to eat comfortably and communicate clearly.

Improved overall health:

Oral health and general health are closely related. Untreated dental issues, especially gum disease, have been linked to a higher chance of developing systemic illnesses like heart disease, diabetes, lung infections, and unfavorable pregnancy outcomes. You can contribute to greater general health and well-being by treating dental problems as soon as they arise.

Enhanced appearance and self-confidence:

Dental issues can have an aesthetic impact on your smile, which can cause self-consciousness and decrease self-confidence. These issues can be resolved with prompt treatment, strengthening your self-esteem and the appearance of your teeth.

To identify any dental issues early, it's crucial to keep up with routine checkups. Additionally, maintaining proper oral hygiene through consistent brushing, flossing, and a healthy diet might aid in preventing the emergence of dental problems.

Consult with a dental expert right away if you suffer any dental pain, sensitivity, swelling, or other unsettling symptoms. They can assess your condition, administer the proper care, and avert more problems. Keep in mind that early intervention is essential for preserving excellent oral health and avoiding later, more serious dental issues.

Conclusion

Keeping good dental hygiene is crucial for your general health and a healthy smile.

You may prevent dental problems, promote fresh breath, and support ideal oral health by adhering to the advised oral hygiene routines and guidelines, such as consistent brushing, flossing, and mouthwash use.

A healthy mouth is further supported by minimizing sugar-sweetened foods and beverages, eating a balanced diet, and drinking lots of water.
Keep in mind to schedule routine cleanings and exams at the dentist.

You can benefit from a confident smile and long-term dental health by prioritizing oral hygiene.